In this case, you can't judge a book by its cover...

Chronicles of the Chronically Ill

Mind-blowing stories of unimaginable struggle that resulted in extraordinary strength

Jai Publishing
WRITE. RELEASE. HEAL.

Scripture quotations taken from the Holy Bible, King James Version.

Printed in the United States of America

ISBN-13: 978-0692157084

ISBN-10: 0692157085

Contents

Foreword

By Jamie Hopkins
Author, Publisher & Victim's Advocate

In 2009, I was diagnosed with ilionguinal nerve neuropathy—an injured nerve in simple terms. Prior to that diagnosis, I had been experiencing a sharp needle-like pain in my lower pelvic area for about six years! Yep, it took doctors six freaking years to diagnose my pain. And it wasn't until I decided to search for a doctor who specialized in nerve pain that I was finally diagnosed. Hundreds of doctors appointments, two failed surgeries, and thousands of dollars later, I was told from the specialist that not just one, but two major nerves were damaged during that surgery back in 2003 to remove a cyst on my right ovary.

In case you're not familiar with how ilionguinal nerve neuropathy feels, imagine inserting the largest needle you can find into your private area. Yeah, it's excruciating pain. And since the diagnosis, it appeared as if my pain got worse. I was on antidepressants back then, which were the only medications for nerve pain. And I was getting regular steroid shots that cost almost $1,000 a piece, with medical insurance! I did mention he was a specialist, right? Yeah, he was expensive, but he made the pain go away. I would pay anything for relief! And I did. I had to get a series of steroid shots in my pelvic area five consecutive days for one week annually. And I continued this practice of getting the annual steroid shots ($5,000 out of pocket) until I could no longer afford it. When I lost my job three years later, I lost my insurance and my financial access to these steroid shots.

Sitting too long, walking too far, lifting heavy items, and my monthly period are all triggers to the inflammation. Just recently, I realized that anxiety is not my friend either. The anxiety inflames the nerve, and the nerve pain provokes the anxiety. So they bounce off of each other, causing a discomfort you won't believe. THIS is my life, my new normal. But because you can't see it, many believe I'm as healthy as it comes. I get funny looks when I can barely walk or ask for help to lift a box.

Just as I had to find a way to cope with my diagnosis, and refuse to allow my new normal to prevent me from living and enjoying life (it was a decision), these authors have done that and so much more! When you read this book, you will feel their pain, you will see their struggles, but you will also rejoice in their truth: there is life beyond the diagnosis!

Ultimately, it comes down to this: you can either give in to the pain, as much as it sucks, OR you can choose to press through it, as much as it sucks. These authors have made the bold decision to live in spite of their physical and mental limitations. They found a way to do it. And if they can do it, I hope it gives you hope to know that you can too! All it takes is a decision to fight, because you are not in this war alone.

Did you know?

It is estimated that at least 1.5 million Americans live with **LUPUS**. People who suffer with lupus may experience painful joints, extreme fatigue, hair loss, cognitive issues, and physical impairments that affect every area of their lives.[1]

"It is happening. I trust the process!" - Dr. Marquita S. Blades

~ CHAPTER ONE ~

You Don't Look Sick!

BY DR. MARQUITA S. BLADES

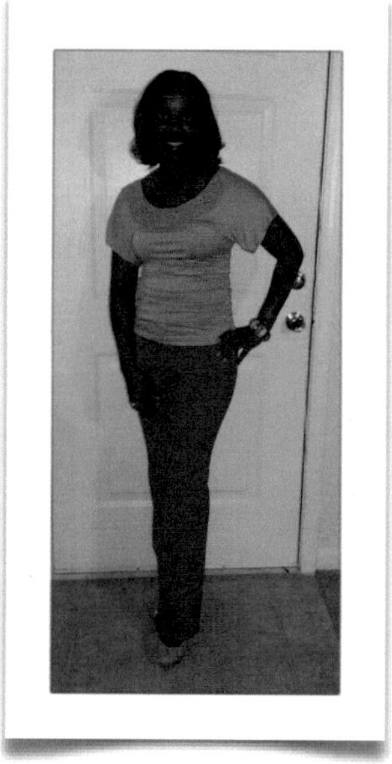

There's a story behind this picture… five years ago, I had just moved into this 1-bedroom apartment in Griffin, Georgia with my mom as my full-time caregiver. My lupus was out of control. I was taking Celebrex, methotrexate, plaquinel, prednisone, and was being prepped for the weekly Enbrel injection by getting the shingles vaccine, which, by the way, my body was unable to build immunity against.

But WHY was this case? My home was in foreclosure after having been fired from a teaching position that I hated (I was truly happy about that part), leaving me to work in a low-paying school district earning 15K less than what I had previously been making. This district had made massive cuts and they didn't credit me for all of my years of experience.

Rather than save the home, I wanted to finish my doctorate. I was already five years in at this point and tuition would cost me about $1300 per month on an institutional payment plan; which was twice the amount of my mortgage. I was also coming out of a relationship that had turned physically violent. One time was all it took for me—the way my lupus was set up, I didn't have time to be getting beat on, besides, I was not created to be a punching bag.

SIDE NOTE: Ladies, please stop taking abuse. JUST LEAVE! Now, back to my life...

My life was completely upside down at 35 years old. I felt as if I was moving backwards and none of the accomplishments I'd achieved up to that point mattered. But I looked good, right? Humph! You never know what a person is going through. You also can't let your circumstances define you. Dig deep. Find a way. If you can't find a way, make one! My situation got a lot worse before it got better. I've chronicled my journey with chronic illness, lupus, to be exact. Let the chronicles begin…

The Pre-Lupus Chronicles

I've always seen myself being a lot of things, but sick was not one of them. Of course, it is always a possibility, but it is not something that you really think will happen to you. When you make plans for your life, you don't factor in time to deal with an illness. "I think around 33 years old, I'll get a disease. Not sure what type or which one yet, but I do want to just make note of the fact that I'll be getting one", said no one EVER!

So no, I did not see this coming, but I can distinctly remember the morning that I realized that something was seriously wrong with me. It was different from any other time that I'd felt that something was wrong. I was in pain. I could not move. I'd been in pain before where I had difficulty moving, but this time, I absolutely could not move. No matter how many times my brain told my arms to bend, they wouldn't budge. For a brief moment, I thought that this was the beginning of something that, as my grandmamma used to say, "Ajax couldn't take off." Thankfully, I'd slept with my phone next to me, so I called my mama to come help me. She massaged me up, got me moving, we speculated causes, and I went on about my business.

At that time, it wasn't far-fetched for me to be in this type of pain. I worked out with a trainer five days per week, I danced at a studio three days a week, I was a member of a Liturgical Dance ministry, I was teaching full-time and frequently attended after school events. Weekends were mine for the taking. I had an active social and dating life. Finally, it was nothing for me to jump on a plane or hop in my car for a quick getaway. This pain event was memorable, but I certainly did not think it would change my life in all of the ways that it did.

After another couple of episodes like this I became serious about finding some answers. Six months, several specialists, and hours of research later, I had lupus. Finally, a name. Now what? Deny, deny, deny! At that time I was an avid church-goer and one of the main tenets of the black church in particular is to just not "claim" any adversity. In essence, it is an ill-placed faith that teaches you to act in denial because God has everything under control. BIGGEST. MISTAKE. OF. MY. LIFE. This attitude allowed my lupus to fester. And fester, it did.

Now, I'm not blaming the church, but I am illustrating the point of the attitude I had at that time when I believed that I needed the church to find the answers to the questions that I had in life – but that's for another anthology! Let's get back to the chronicles…

First Came the Pain

Initially, pain was my only symptom. It was plenty. You see, it wasn't "take a Tylenol" pain. It was "go to the doctor NOW" pain. Thankfully, I had not overlooked the important aspect of selecting a rheumatologist. I selected one of the best in Georgia. I did aaaallll the research and I was ready. When I started having pain, all I had to do was call her up and she'd give me something to take. I took it. The pain went away. I resumed activities. Simple enough, right? Wrong.

This routine became a vicious cycle that over time required more and stronger meds in order to control the same level of pain. I was really shocked to realize how much time I spent in and out of my rheumatologist's office rather than actually living life. Whenever I'd ask about any therapies to help keep me out of pain, she seemed to be irritated. All she wanted to talk about was medicines and dosages. She wasn't at all interested in talking about anything else I could do to manage my illness like diet, exercise, or natural supplements.

Eventually, I'd fire her, but that took too many years and far too many doses to come about. For the time being, my pain was bad, but it was nothing that would stop me. This will be significant later.

Then Came Even More Pain

This time, it wasn't tolerable. This time I couldn't just take something and make it go away. This time, I could not work through it when it didn't go away. I mean, it lasted for days even. My rheumatologist started giving me steroid injections. They worked like you wouldn't believe and they lasted for a good while too. I thought I was winning because now I could work a stretch of time without having to take any days off and, in my mind, my lupus would not really be affecting me.

The frequency of the steroid shots increased, but at the time, they were a means to an end and I could get them whenever I needed them. This problem was not a problem at all. I was beginning to take on the mentality that there was medication for everything and if I just followed the regimen, I'd be fine to continue living my life.

But here's the part I haven't told you yet. At this point, my pain had caused me to give up some of the activities that I had previously enjoyed. For years, I had been a member of the dance ministry at my church. It was my absolute favorite thing. The dance ministry had allowed me to live out my dream of really learning to dance. You see, I'd always wanted to take dance lessons as a child, but it wasn't possible. Joining the dance ministry allowed me to learn the ballet, jazz, and modern technique that I'd admired of other dancers for years. And I was GOOD!

But, I'd given dance up around 2012 because the aftermath of rehearsals and performances had taken a toll on me. The soreness and stiffness that came after a rehearsal made it difficult for me to work some days. Or, if it wasn't the soreness and stiffness, the sheer fatigue would slow me down or completely stop me in my tracks. I usually had to take off work the day after a performance because we did two in a day and the trifecta of soreness, stiffness, and fatigue would immediately claim me.

I'd also given up working out consistently. Prior to my diagnosis and earlier into it, I worked out with a personal trainer at 4:30 a.m., 5 days per week. Y'all I was finer than frog hair back then! Not only did I look good, but I was fit and strong. This helped me to be a better dancer. I had tons of energy, so my teaching was always on point. Not to sound like a sales pitch for a workout plan, but all of the benefits of working out, I could see firsthand. So you can imagine how hard it was for me to give this up.

I didn't just stop cold turkey. I saw my performance tapering off and my pain and fatigue increasing, so over time it went from 5 days to 3, then 1, until eventually, I just wasn't working out anymore. Slowly the pieces of me that made me "me" were being pulled from my grasp and I didn't even realize how much of myself I was losing.

Also, by this time, the wonderful and loving guy I had been dating and was planning a future with decided that he could "find someone better" for whom he did not have to be "a nurse" and abruptly ended our relationship. I was surprised! He had never expressed any frustrations prior to this point, and I thought that I'd done a good job of not allowing my illness to impact him… I mean, as much as had been possible.

I was hurt, but in all honesty, I didn't have time to worry about him. My house was also in foreclosure. This was partially circumstance and partially a conscious decision that I'd made. When I was fired the year before and regained employment, I could have chosen to catch up my mortgage in spite of being severely underpaid. I wanted my doctoral degree more. I had put pursuit of my degree on hold because I realized I was having a hard time concentrating and processing information. It had started to take me twice as long to research information and three times as long to read and process it. Writing papers, something that I could previously do with my eyes closed, had now become a challenge as well. I wasn't as sharp or efficient as I had previously been.

Add to this that my joints were often swollen and in pain. Some days I simply could not move my fingers to press the keys on my laptop, so I told myself to take some time off and come back to it. The way I saw it, I had experienced homeownership, but I had not yet experienced holding the title of doctor. Getting my PhD (I actually decided on an EdD) had been a goal of mine since high school. There was no way I was going to hold on to all of those credits I'd earned and not finish, so rather than focusing on catching up the mortgage, I chose to pay the balance I owed my university and re-enroll in my program. Here was another thing (taking time off from my EdD program) that I had given up although in my mind lupus wasn't really impacting my life.

If you are familiar with the foreclosure process, you know it takes a long time. I also kept applying for assistance programs which delayed it even longer. In essence, I was squatting in my own home, trying to figure out what I was going to do. I was terribly ill and losing more and more of my independence by the day. I didn't have the income I had once enjoyed and I desperately wanted to finish my degree. I knew I had issues comprehending and synthesizing information but I would cross that bridge when I got to it.

When that school year ended, I decided to continue in my summer position that I'd had for years (managing national STEM programs for high school students) because I really needed the money. It was hard on me because running programs with upwards of 400 students and 30 staff members requires a lot of work, but because I had years of experience doing it, I was able to somehow make it happen. During that summer, I met a guy. We dated. It was great. He was ready. It got serious.

Then Went My Voice

The first major occurrence, aside from pain, that I had with my lupus was developing polyps on my vocal cords. That fall, once school started back, I noticed that I would easily lose my voice every day. Being that I was a teacher, you can understand how this quickly became a problem. The polyps weren't cancerous and could be lasered off so that's what I did. No big deal. This lupus thing still wasn't really affecting me.

During this time of having vocal cord surgery, I thought I had found another great relationship, except this time, my illness would not be a problem. This guy seemed to get it and not hold it against me. What I did not know is that he had issues of his own and he was tracking my every move. No, I mean really tracking my every move. Apparently, while I was sick, he had taken the liberty of putting spyware on my laptop and phone that allowed him to listen to all of my voicemails, read all of my emails, and even receive my phone calls at the same time that I was receiving them.

By this time, my ex, the one who did not want to be my nurse, was contacting me, as he had realized that he may have made a mistake. New guy was reading these messages unbeknownst to me. I actually never responded to a single message (I'm a one and done kind of person), because I knew I had no interest, but I guess new guy missed that part. Trouble was brewing behind the scenes and I no idea that any of this was going on.

One night while at his home, it all "came to a head" as my mama would say. I was taking a shower and when I stepped out and turned around he was so close to my face that we were close enough to kiss but still had enough space between us for me to realize that this was not a romantic encounter. My heart started to race. I was scared and confused. What was going on? I mean we had just baked some cookies before I went into the shower. He started yelling about "m—f—s" always calling and emailing me and named one in particular… a friend that I've had for almost 20 years! A friend that is married and that he'd met multiple times. They were supposed to be cool!

He was standing in my face and started poking and pushing me backwards as he recited verbatim the conversations that I'd had with this friend. Again, I was scared and confused. How did he know any of this? I tried to get around him and was yelling at him to get out of my face. My joints were inflamed. My muscles were weak. I'd lost my upper body strength to lupus a long time ago. Not that I could have overtaken him anyway, but I was completely incapable of defending myself. What was I going to do?

Somehow I made it out of the bathroom and managed to put on a pair of sweatpants. I was trying to get dressed but the yelling and conversation quotes kept coming. Pushes had come to shoves. I kept asking, "what are you talking about?" Not because I didn't know what he was talking about, but because I didn't know how he was able to talk about it. It had not dawned on me that he had been stalking me and in the moment of getting beat up, you really don't think about that kind of thing.

Meanwhile, he is still poking and pushing me. Before I could get a shirt on, he actually grabbed me and threw me against the wall. I knew if I didn't get out then, I might not. I had never seen someone so full of rage, nor had I ever been handled like this by anyone so I was already thinking the worst – he's going to beat me to a pulp or ...

I have no idea how, but I was able to get a shirt on and then I went for my phone to call the police. Of course, he took the phone away from me and threw it. It went under the bed and in between being slammed against the wall; I dove for the floor to try to get under the bed to get it. No such luck. He kicked me as I tried to crawl to the edge of the bed and I just knew that it would get much worse.

I managed to get up and spotted my purse on the dresser. I went into the closet with him close on heels still pushing me. I was able to slip my feet into some shoes. All the while he is still ranting and raving about me being sneaky and not keeping it "a hunned" (that's 100, as in 100%, as in being totally honest); that I should have told him every time someone called me but he had to find out on his own and now I was making him act this way.

He turned around and left the closet and I knew that was my chance. I ran out of the closet, grabbed my purse, and made a dash down the hallway past the bedrooms in which his children had been during this entire episode. Of course he ran after me. I made it outside, into my car, and locked the door in just enough time to miss the large glob of spit that he fired at me. I drove off, straight to the nearest police station. They escorted me back to his house for my belongings and that was the night I regained my voice. The rest of my lupus symptoms, however, were not so manageable after that incident. In fact, they only got worse.

The Medication Chronicles

After officially putting my home on the market for short sale, I was told I'd have to stop squatting in it, so I packed up my belongings and moved back to my hometown of Griffin, Georgia. This would make it easier for my mom to help me. She'd been my full-time caregiver for about eight months or so already, but she was also back and forth between mine and my brother's house. I didn't like that, so I decided to just go there. Also, it was only a seven mile difference from my job in the opposite direction.

I was still determined to complete my degree so I only took a one-bedroom apartment for my mama and me to share so that I could still afford my tuition. I could barely pay for everything but somehow each month, between my part-time and contract work, my mama and I made it. She did the household chores, grocery shopping, and physically helped me take care of myself, and I went to work and collected a check. She even graded papers for me so I could work on my dissertation on the weekends and in evenings.

Sometimes, I slept the entire weekend because the pain and fatigue of working all week had overcome me. As soon as I would accumulate a sick day, I'd use it. I so wanted to quit my job. Not because I hated it but because I could no longer do it the way that it needed to be done. I felt terrible going to work and not being on fire to teach, but rather being on fire from inflammation and pain. My students could tell the difference, but they gave me grace because they liked me. I was completely miserable and the merry-go-round of medications that I would soon be riding only multiplied it.

From early 2013 to early 2014, I was on a combination of all of the following: Celebrex, plaquinel, tramadol, prednisone, and methotrexate (which is a low dose chemotherapy drug). None of it made me feel better. I was still in pain most of the time and needed assistance with almost everything physical. Don't ask me how I was holding a job. Because none of this was really working, I was still going in every 4-6 weeks to get steroid shots that didn't even last the full 4-6 weeks. They were only working for about 3 weeks at the most, but I was willing to take any bit of relief that I could get.

After much debate and research, I decided to take a chance on the weekly Enbrel injection. I needed something to believe in. It just had to work! Before I could get it, I had to have already had the shingles vaccine, which of course, at 35 years old, I had not. Shingles is an "old people's" disease. If you're wondering what would make a 35-year-old with a compromised immune system take any vaccine, then you and I are on the same page. Even today, I can't tell you how I fixed my mind to think that this was the right move to make. The only thing I can offer is that I truly was desperate and I just needed something to give me enough hope so that I could make it another day.

It was getting so that I did not want to get out of bed in the mornings and I'd cry myself all the way to work on the mornings that my mama didn't drive me. I felt sorry for myself and I was willing to do anything that I thought would change my situation, even if it meant taking a risk with a vaccine.

As you may have guessed, or as I told you in the beginning of this story, my body did not build up the immunity to shingles. YES... you are looking at, or imagining the face of, a 40-year-old woman who has shingles, but I digress.

I took the vaccine and was able to get the Enbrel injection. I will admit, at first, I saw some improvement. Enough improvement that I could shower on my own, drive myself to work more, and even go out for dinner with friends after work. Something was finally working. I threw myself into my dissertation, determined to finish by the end of 2013; a goal that I ultimately did not meet.

I also started dating again and this time it was really different. We got married! At the end of that same year, 2014, I completed my doctoral program as well. I was still taking my Enbrel and life was moving along. Then one day the Enbrel stopped working and suddenly my husband had traded places with my mama as my caregiver. It was so unfair, I thought. After everything I'd been through, why couldn't I just have a piece of a normal life again? Why couldn't my husband have a whole wife who could be a fully active partner?

After another long cycle of constant pain, frequent steroid shots, daily steroid pills along with other pills that I can't even remember, and the weekly injection—all with little to no relief—my husband and I decided enough was enough. A new school year had started and I'd already missed three days by the third week. I was already crying every morning before I could even leave the house. To top that off, I'd learned that between the frequent steroid shots and daily steroid use, my bones were showing signs of early onset osteoporosis. I wasn't even 40 yet and I was already showing signs of another "old people's" disease.

We decided it was time for me to resign and take a different approach to my health, but even that was not as easy as I thought it would be. I'd need medical documentation in order to avoid any penalties for breaking my teaching contract and to prevent any attempts to revoke my teaching license. Although I was leaving teaching in the classroom, I still very much valued my license and did not want it being revoked over something like this.

So, I went to my rheumatologist so she could complete the paperwork. I just knew I'd have her support after seeing me struggle for so many years but I was as wrong as two left shoes. She was the total opposite—combative and defensive—and told me that I could, in fact, continue working because she had seen me "work in worse conditions that this".

While the "Quita" in me wanted to curse her out, all I could do was cry. It was like this nightmare was never going to end. I knew I couldn't continue as I had been for the past couple of years and it was clear I did not have her support. I told you before that she was never interested in anything but prescriptions… it had not dawned on me before, but she was never interested in my healing, she just wanted me and my laundry list of prescriptions on her patient roster.

I didn't know what to do at this point, but my husband reassured me that we had made the right decision regarding me exiting the classroom, so I moved forward. (Just so you know, my teaching license is still intact.)

It's been two years since I resigned from teaching. I have been med-free for a year and half – following a holistic regimen—and I have not been in constant pain every single day. There have been some bad days for sure, but nothing like it used to be!

A portion of this chapter was typed from a hospital bed, during a 9-day stay, as I recovered from my first major lupus flare in almost two years. I've got some major work to do to make sure this thing stays in remission, but I know it can be done! There are still so many things that I can't do without assistance on some days like: turning a doorknob, brushing my teeth, anything involving my hair, taking a shower and getting dressed, putting on lotion, working out, driving, carrying my purse, cooking and cleaning, or just getting up and walking. These are things that most people do without thinking about but I don't have that luxury. I do have to think about every physical action I take and what impact it will have on the next. I have to make conscious decisions about how I want to use the small amount of mobility and range of motion I have in order to get the most of my days.

Looking cute? Can't do that without help. I can't fasten buttons and I can no longer zip dresses with zippers in the back. I can barely get a blazer on sometimes. That eliminates about 75% of my options for clothing. I have to meticulously plan what clothes I can wear on what days based on whether or not there will be someone (my husband or mama) available to help me get it on and get it fastened. (This is also why my husband travels with me to all speaking engagements, so I can look the part and represent myself in the best way possible).

I used to be hard on people about their appearances until I couldn't maintain my own. It was so easy to look at a person and wonder, "why did she come out looking like that?". Now, my first thought when someone is not put together is, "I wonder what she had to go through to make it out of the house today."

There have been days when all I could do was throw something on and limp my way through the day. There were days when I knew my hair was disheveled, feet were ashy, and my clothes were wrinkled (the iron is too heavy to pick up sometimes), but I had no choice. You'd be surprised at how quickly you get over yourself when you need to perform simple, everyday tasks, yet can't.

I've had to call and ask colleagues to come and let me out of a restroom stall because I couldn't twist the knob and strangers have had to take off and replace my gas cap because I was just too weak to do it myself. When you look normal and have to ask for that type of help, you don't get a friendly yes... people get agitated or ignore you completely, but what are you supposed to do? Other teachers, male for that matter, have watched me limp and struggle to pull my rolling bag to my classroom and have not offered an ounce of assistance because in their minds, I didn't look sick!

Forget about an active social and community life. 70% of the plans I make get cancelled if I don't either have someone to help me get ready to go or drive me to the event. I typically can't do both and still have energy for the remainder of that day or the next day. It's just easier to stay home. Visiting people or riding their cars? Child, please! I need to be in a warm temperature at all times—most people like to be cool. For this reason, I don't like going to anyone's home, especially not for extended visits. I end up freezing to death and hurting the entire time.

I drink everything room temperature so that the coolness of the glass does not cause my Raynaud's to flare up. This is a side-condition, if you will, that causes your extremities to lose circulation, turn purple, and go numb. If I touch a cold soda can or glass, I can expect to have numb, purple fingers for at least 30-40 minutes. Sometimes they don't go all the way numb though, and I get to have a little pain too.

I could go on, but I think you understand and I know you're wondering, "exactly how does all of this constitute a win?" Well, I'll tell you the story of the pink dress.

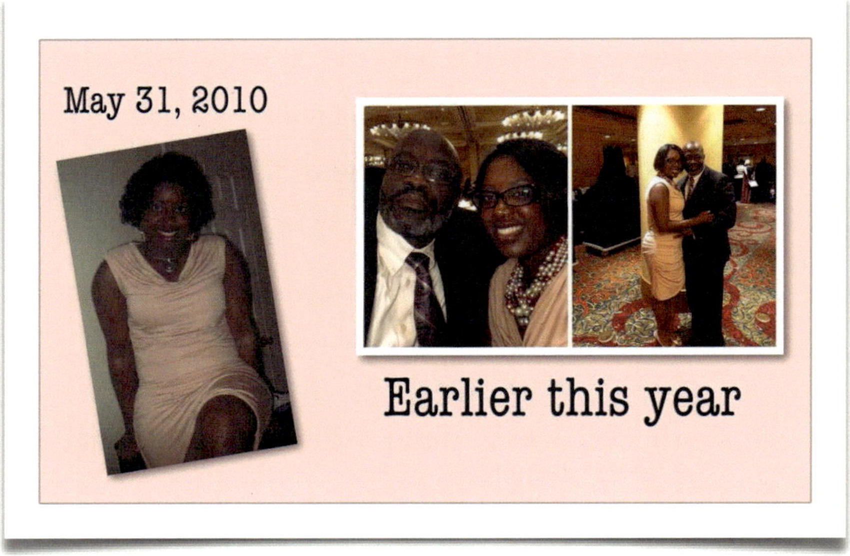

The Pink Dress

[Facebook memories always cause me to reflect. The picture above recently came up in my Facebook memories.]

In 2010, I had dreams of doing what I do now, but I had no reason to pursue my dream of being a leader in science education, an author, and speaker. I was living what I perceived to be my best life. I was earning more than enough money to support my lifestyle, had a lovely townhome, and was actively dating. I was involved in the community and had a great social life. I was teaching in a great school and loved my students! Why would I give up the stability that I created FOR AND BY myself for something I wasn't even sure I could do? Oh, that pink dress fit me so well!

Fast forward to 2018. I AM a leader in science education, an author, and speaker. I'm no longer dating; I'm married to an outstanding partner who supports my growth. Were it not for a series of shakedowns in my career (getting fired), my finances (losing my home), my dating life (I was physically assaulted), and my health (lupus turned all the way up); I would have never had a reason to make faith moves.

Yeah, the pink dress LOOKED better on me THEN, but I'm WEARING it better NOW. #TrustTheProcess

Did you know?

EPILEPSY is NOT as rare as one may think. In fact, studies show that there are more than twice as many people with epilepsy in the U.S. as the number of people with cerebral palsy, muscular dystrophy, multiple sclerosis, and cystic fibrosis COMBINED.[2]

"Staying vulnerable is a risk we have to take if we want to experience connection." - Brené Brown

~ Chapter Two ~

It's Not All In My Head

By Sarah Beth Wright

Epilepsy seems to be a scary word to many, myself included. Going through life, I have tried to avoid the discussion or knowledge of my neurological diagnosis to others. A fear of judgment due to people not being able to physically see what is included in my diagnosis, and the insecurity of people questioning my ability to be me—wife, mom, teacher, and more. I have come to realize epilepsy is a tremendous part of who I am. Owning this and showing others how it has affected, and continues to affect my life everyday is my goal.

* * * *

In 1995, as a 14-year-old girl, I stood at the top of the hill straddling my bicycle – my brain was in a fog. My brother and sister stood at the bottom of the hill with my mom waving and shouting, "Come on Sarah! What are you doing?"

I slowly walked my bike down the hill to my mom. She automatically sensed things were not normal. "Are you okay?" She asked with concern. My words could not come out as I needed them to, and describing what just happened could not take place at the time.

Over the next month, similar situations happened. They seemed to become more frequent and more intense. My parents were very active, and had me in to see my pediatrician. After several tests, we were told I was having seizures. My doctor placed me on medication to control the seizures, however the medicine did not control the issues. Being that my seizures continued, and I began having other symptoms so my parents pushed for an MRI, a magnetic resonance imaging scan of my brain.

My mom held my hand as we walked into the lobby of the hospital. She said a prayer with me, and looked at me with a concerned face. With strength, she stated, "No matter what the MRI shows, we will get through this." As a young teenager, I was oblivious to the seriousness of the pending results. I was just a kid for crying out loud!

After the MRI scan and leaving the doctor's office, we decided to eat lunch at our favorite Chinese restaurant. As we finished eating, they brought out our fortune cookies. I cracked open mine and read it like I always did. I was expecting to life like usual, however when I started to read the words, they came out in slow motion, "You are about to face a life changing event." Mom and I stared at each other for a few seconds, and then changed the subject. At that moment, I knew we would be getting a call soon.

That evening, my doctor called my parents with the news we feared. The MRI had shown a brain tumor. Various emotions took over the family in the dining room as we prayed and cried together. Although we had an answer, a large amount of unknown fear had just entered into our lives. We wanted an answer to the episodes I was having; we needed an answer; but never in our wildest dreams did we think THAT would be the answer! A brain tumor at fourteen.

Walking into school the next day, the diverse feelings of fear, nervousness, insecurity, and confidence bounced through my head throughout the day. My life would now be different than those students surrounding me. My biggest fear—were they going to shave my head?

* * * *

On December 19, 1995, the doctors performed brain surgery to remove the tumor. This procedure, along with continued medication, helped control my seizures. When I went into surgery my parents were given warnings of many neurological changes that could take place. They made contact with speech and occupational therapists, everything would be prepared when I needed the assistance.

Coming out of surgery, I appeared to be myself. I seemed to walk and talk like always. We were blessed with an amazing group of people at Arkansas Children's Hospital that I still remember today by name and face. I will always remember celebrating my 15th Christmas in the hospital bed, and realizing my life was good. The surgery was successful, and I was going home. I learned at an early age my life was a blessing.

* * * *

As a child, scores ranked me very high in my class. My test scores were always grades above where I was actually at the time. After my first epileptic episode, I struggled in regular classes. When I read books, I felt like the words blew through my brain without sticking. My favorite subject of reading had become my least favorite because of my struggle to comprehend.

Innocently family and friends began referring to me as an airhead, not knowing why I could not always catch on to what was going on quickly or remember what had happened in a situation I had learned about before. I felt on guard and sometimes defensive. Many times I felt I needed to prove myself. Throughout high school, I became insecure in this area.

As my life continued, I began to realize the differences other people were not able to see. My brain needed more rest than others. Making myself nap became the norm. Many times thoughts would be in my head, however I was unable to complete a sentence because my words would not come out smoothly. Finding words to match what I am trying to say could throw an awkward pause in a conversation.

Two days before my senior graduation, I woke up in the middle of the night to my dad and mom bent over my bed. The shaking bed had awaken my sister. With fright, she woke up my parents and they came quickly to my bedside. Dad said quietly, "Sissy, you're okay, but you had a seizure." My ears could hear his words, however my mouth could not speak to him. Fear was obvious in the room. This was the first time I had a grand mal seizure.

In the past, I had always used this in my defense. I don't have *that* kind of seizure. Laying there afterwards, I realized one of my worst fears had come to light. My body was shaking due to contracted muscles, and I had been unconscious. I now had stepped over to *that* kind of seizure.

Over the next few months I began having grand mal seizures repeatedly. For the safety of myself and others, my driver's license was taken from me. The doctors and my parents were concerned about the unconsciousness during my seizures. If I blacked out while driving I could easily kill myself or someone else.

* * * *

Now being a freshly graduated young adult, my younger 14-year-old sister drove me around quite a bit. I started college that following Fall, and friends and family would help me get to school and work. Friends I had during this time will always be close to my heart. My needs seemed to always fit into their schedules. My husband, who was my boyfriend at the time, made me feel secure. He was concerned and wanted to know the details. My sister had the weight of the world on her shoulders at such an early age, yet still pushed through as one of my biggest advocates.

During that time, though, I felt smothered. As a young adult, independence (the one thing every kid looks forward to) was put on hold. Being left alone was not an option. The seizures began to increase and were taking over my life. When we met with my doctor, he explained scar tissue was causing this reaction and gave me the option of a second surgery. He explained the risks, and my parents allowed me to have a very strong opinion in the choice. Looking forward at my life, I could not imagine not trying this solution.

In January 2000, I went in for my second brain surgery. My fear this time was much stronger. Being older, I was able to process the risks and possible side effects of the surgery taking place. My boyfriend stood beside me through the whole process. I feared I would awaken as a different person after surgery and he would leave. When I opened my eyes after surgery, I recognized Dad standing beside me, and I knew I was okay.

When my doctor released me, I returned home. Within the first year after my second surgery, I had two grand mal seizures. Time passed during this transition where I grieved. I felt confused and angry. I questioned God, and I felt I was being punished. If He is the maker of all things, why did God make me the way I am? Why was I having to go through this heartbreak? What was I doing wrong? If I changed my actions, would the seizures go away?

I since come to realize God does not function that way. But you have to understand that I was so young and had gone through a lot as a result of my brain tumor. Of course I would be emotional and confused, even in my faith in God. Many times in life, situations happen that are part of this world. The experiences make us who we are, however God is not using them against us. Instead, He turns it around for us.

Okay, back to the story! The doctor changed my medication, so the surgery and medicine change were able to control my seizures. My driver's license was given back to me, and I became confident the choice I made to follow through with my second surgery would be good for my life.

* * * *

After I returned home from the hospital, not much time passed before I returned to college. My insecurities with reading began to sneak up on me. Like before, I could read and read and read, yet I was unable to recollect the words I read. I would study before a test, and I would not do well. This became normal, and I grew discouraged. If I shared this with others, I felt the doubt. I think my professors felt like I was a slacker and lazy when it came to school. They did not understand or saw the effort I put into the books. At that time, I guarded myself from the truth. I did not share my diagnosis or medical past with my professors, so they had no way of knowing that I was suffering silently with that secret. I wanted to prove myself to others. And, really I wanted to prove to myself that I could live a *normal* life.

* * * *

When I moved away to a state university, I finally felt freedom. The feeling of being smothered by my parents was no longer strong. I could be me. When I look back at that time, I was in a very large state of denial. I needed help but I was in denial about that just so I could keep my freedom.

Several times my roommate had to come and get me because I was unable to drive due to auras or nausea and dizziness, which was all related to my epilepsy. Holding on to my freedom gave me the feeling of control. Many times I went out of my way to make sure my parents knew nothing about what was really going on. I wanted to live like a college student—have the ability to be up late, make friends, have a crazy schedule, and not feel the side effects.

Putting together the difficulties with learning and my struggles with my health, college became a very frustrating and wearing task. College was a must in my parents' eyes, and goal for my future. I yearned to be a teacher. I continued, and I finished! Reflecting on that time in my life, I realized my college degree was a huge success.

* * * *

Beginning life after college, my boyfriend and I got married. He always joked with me about my 'Sarah naps'. Sleeping twelve hours a day seemed normal to me. As time went on, I realized when I lacked sleep my brain was foggy, and my words became mixed up. I later found that the medical term for this is Dysphasia.

The insecurities of judgment from others always lurked above me. Do they understand why my body and brain needed rest? Do they think I am clueless when we had a conversation? Many times I simply stood back and didn't speak in social situations due to this fear.

In 2006, I became pregnant with our first child. My doctor suggested we see a high-risk obstetrician for the safety of myself and the baby. We followed through with that advice. I continued with my medication, and did my best to follow a sleep schedule. Jacob, our first child, and myself were watched very carefully throughout the 40 weeks. We were grateful my pregnancy was a success.

When Jacob was three months old, I began my career in Education. Teaching students had always been my dream. As a child I would line up teddy bears and Barbie dolls so I could teach them how to read.

When I started my career at my first school, I knew my principal had doubt in my quiet, pushover personality. She learned quickly how I worked with my students. As I whispered in class, the students whispered with me. My first year as a teacher was enlightening as an educator, a parent, and a person still in denial of my neurological diagnosis.

* * * *

As I continued working, being a mom, and a wife, I noticed that my choice of having that second surgery back in the day definitely had it's benefits and ranked high as a must, there were also significant areas of my life affected. That surgery cut out a large piece of my brain. And though it helped with my seizures, I noticed as the years went by that my words continued to get mixed up. I could not keep anything neat. It seemed as if I was numb to chaos. As I noticed these things myself, I wondered if others did also.

When I was pregnant with our second son, I was put on bedrest at 27 weeks. Seizure activity was taking place, and my obstetrician wanted to keep myself and the baby safe. Staying at home was frustrating. Teaching the students in my classroom was where I wanted to be but couldn't. The pregnancy slowly passed, and we were blessed with our second child.

During that time, the stress of daily living with a family began to show through my neuro symptoms. Anytime my children took a nap, I took a nap also. My bedtime was early on weekdays, so I was able to teach my students, care for our kids, and our house, as my husband worked and attended school out of town.

* * * *

Ironically, in the midst of our busy and chaotic lives, my husband had an accident which caused him to have a Traumatic Brain Injury (TBI). Our lives turned upside down. As the wife and mother, I tried to do everything by myself as a caregiver, and I failed. I could feel the questions from those close, watching from the outside. The situation felt very similar to my first year of college. Friends and family were driving my husband everywhere. We had to schedule with other people in order to carry on with our own lives. Here I was back to depending on everyone else for everyday living.

Not long after his accident, my husband began speech, occupational, and physical therapy at a Neurorehab location. As I would sit in and listen to his therapists give me updates on my husband, I took notes for myself. Many of the descriptions they were giving were me! The ability to describe what he wanted to say, but not know the actual word—I do this regularly. My husband was now living my life. Literally.

* * * *

My sister was, and still is, my walking thesaurus. I would text her a description, and she would send me the word. She was aware of this need of mine before I ever accepted it. Getting words jumbled or mixed up. That was the awareness I came to, and when I would mention it, people would respond, "Well, I do that." They didn't really understand what was going on in my head.

My first grade class finished sentences for me. They would make the comment, lovingly, as they carried me along the way, "Mrs. Wright's got her words mixed up again." I am indebted to the grace of children.

My third pregnancy went extremely smooth. My doctor had me on half the dosage I was normally on, and there were no problems arising when it came to my seizures. After his birth, denial crept in, and I began to think, maybe I can quit taking my medicine and all of this will be fine. Such a foolish decision!! I learned very quickly nothing had gone away. My brain is wired the way it is. There is nothing I can do to change that.

* * * *

As our life continued as a family, I watched my children, my husband, and those around us grow with me in knowledge when it comes to the brain. In many ways, our life is based around our brains. In the Wright family, we have to put a little extra attention in that area daily. There are simple things the boys know that keeps Mom safe. Do not flash lights in her eyes. She's going to need her nap, and so does Daddy these days because of his injury. They fill in the missing words, which sometimes can be a bonus because their vocabulary is much higher than mine.

I have learned what seems like organization to me, can be chaos to others. My brain is not organized like before, so taking time to truly organize areas of life physically is wearing to me mentally. Although others are able to plan ahead and be prepared, I perform best doing things as I go. If I prepare ahead, most of the items are forgotten or wasted because I do not recall what I planned to use them for. I am very aware this can come across as flighty or unprepared. However, that is not the case. Not in MY case.

Although my relationship with neurology began when I was 14-years-old, I just accepted the reality of my diagnosis this past year. Using the word *epilepsy* always had a tone I did not want to hear. Owning my childhood illness and how it has affected my entire life helped me accept who I am. Many times the idea that I had a brain tumor seemed surreal—a story from a book. However going through that experience made me the person I am today.

Epilepsy is not easy. Communicating with others after two brain surgeries is frustrating at times. In contrary to the previous, I am here. I am alive. God gave me the ability to be a wife, a mom, a teacher, and to share my story. This is my journey.

Did you know?

LUPUS is 2-3 times more likely to affect women of color—African Americans, Hispanics/Latinos, Asians, Native Americans, Alaska Natives, Native Hawaiians and other Pacific Islanders. 1 out of 537 of African American women have lupus.[3]

"To be sick and not know that you are sick is the worst kind of sick." - Dr. Sheva Quinn

~ Chapter Three ~

Homeschooling with Post-Traumatic Stress Disorder (PTSD) and Lupus

By Dr. Sheva Quinn

I can recall standing at the top of the stairs and thinking, "I wonder what would happen if I throw this baby down the stairs." And then something happened, it was like a blanket of peace covered me and told me to go and put the baby down. And so, I went into my room, laid in the bed with my baby, just holding her and rocking her... and both of us crying for four hours straight, until we fell asleep. That next morning, I got up and dressed us both then left out the house to get on with our day, the same as we did every day before. But only this time, after I dropped the baby off at childcare, I went and checked myself into the mental hospital. And yes, I was scared as hell!

I was scared because I had almost 20 years in the military and I didn't know how going to the mental health hospital was going to affect my life and career, but in the end, I knew that I didn't want to kill my crying baby and that I needed some help. I remember being anxious to talk to the doctor and tell them what I was going through, but the paperwork, oh my goodness, I could not get through the paperwork. Each question on the forms just made me cry even more! I guess it was normal because there were boxes of tissues sitting in each and every chair.

Those questions... the more questions I answered, the more I realized that I had been sick almost all of my life; I just didn't know I was sick. Hell, I was even raised by people that were sick.

Finally, I made it back to see a doctor, only to go over in greater detail every question on the forms that I had already answered. And by this time, I cried so much that I didn't have another tear to give… at least so I thought. I started crying a river again! I had broken pieces of tissue all over my face and snot all over my hands, but yet I felt totally numb on the inside. The doctor eventually informed me that I had Post-Traumatic Stress Disorder (PTSD), postpartum depression and I was bipolar. I had no idea of what all that meant. But I did know that I just wanted the doctor to fix the problem. And here it is, almost 10 years later, and the problem still isn't fixed. In fact, when we add a second child, a divorce and lupus to the cocktail, I have to admit that the illnesses have gotten worse and I am just all kind of screwed.

* * * *

The first time I married the father of my children, yes I said the first time, I was in my mid-twenties. And it was tough. It was tough because we were very young and we had no idea of how to be married, nor did we have any role models to follow. Therefore, I would spend all my time in school, trying to get a good education and he would spend all his time hanging out with the boys. After seven years of arguing and fussing about the same issues over and over again, the marriage finally ended.

After being divorced for almost four years, we remarried and moved to England. Shortly after being in England, I became pregnant with our first child and the arguing started back again. I had very little support from my husband while I was pregnant. But I wanted my marriage and my family to work so I assumed that everything was my fault and tried even harder to be a "good" wife. No matter what I did, it wasn't good enough.

Of course, I talked with my psychologist about my marriage and she suggested that I bring my husband in with me on a counseling session. He declined and I continued to suffer and deal with my issues all alone.

Six months after having my first child, I found out that I was pregnant with my second child. Therefore, I did not take prescription meds for my diagnosed illness because it could've affected the birth of the second baby. So here I was, with three mental illnesses, a crying baby, pregnant again, a husband that didn't give a damn, and a failing career. I was literally going crazy!

After I had the second child, I was eligible for retirement from the military, so I applied for retirement and once it was approved, I packed up my children, left my husband and returned to the United States.

When I left England, I left with the understanding that my husband would be retiring the following year and that he would be coming to Georgia to be with me and the children. Well that didn't happen, in fact I moved out and his girlfriend moved in. Later, after being back in the United States, struggling as a broke Air Force veteran with three mental illnesses, two babies, and an unfaithful husband, I filed for a divorce.

As if being unsupportive and unfaithful during the marriage wasn't enough, after I filed for divorce, my ex-husband moved his girlfriend to Georgia and sat her funky ass right here in front of me and the children. But hey, who has time to be hurt when you got two babies to raise? So, I did what I knew how to do, I mentally blocked her out of my head and only dealt with him on co-parenting issues. Still to this day, I haven't dealt with the loss of our marriage. But again, who has time to cry over spilled milk?

* * * *

And for sure, the milk was spilling over! Shortly after my second divorce from the same man, I found out I had lupus. And I can't lie, because I still wanted my family to work… yes, even through all of the bullshit and adultery, I still wanted my family together. I wanted to break generational curses and raise my children in a two-parent household. And for some crazy reason, I thought that my ex-husband would magically care enough to come home and help me raise our children, restore our family. Uh, yeah right, that was so not the case!

I can recall standing in my garage with my eyes full of tears, trying not to let my kids see me cry, and trying to tell him that I was dying. He didn't even hug me or try to console me. I am still trying to figure out was it because he just didn't give a damn or was it because he didn't know how… either way I went through it alone and had no one to hug or console me. Like damn, I am dying and I still can't get a hug from your ass. Had me thinking that he had already wished that my ass was dead. However, it was in that moment that I realized that the marriage was certainly over, as if it wasn't before, and that I had to fight this battle of lupus alone.

After six months of secretly hiding out in my bathroom for private cry sessions and pity parties, I finally got up the nerve to deal with lupus. And once I started to deal with it, my life started to make sense to me. My PTSD and postpartum depression were induced by the lupus. And the reason my muscles felt so weak and my bones ached all the time was, again, because of the lupus. My extreme fatigue was all due to the lupus.

Although I feared dying too young and leaving my children without a mother, I was glad to finally had some answers as to why I always felt like shit and had to take caffeine pills to get on with my day. My fatigue was so bad that I would literally have to pull over on the side of the road and take a nap. There were many times I would be driving two hours away for school, leaving at 4 o'clock in the morning with just me and my girls in the car, and I would have to pull into a restaurant parking lot just to take a 15-minute nap before I could go any further. It was horrible! Even going on short errands around town would exhaust me and I would have to pull over to take naps.

Because my muscles were weak, I would fall down all the time. I even fell three times while pregnant with my children. And the doctors would tell me to be careful and give me braces to wear on my knees... it was the lupus! Looking back and now knowing the symptoms, I believe that I had lupus for at least 7 to 10 years before I was even diagnosed. In fact, I know I had lupus while I was pregnant with my children.

Thus far, the hardest part about living with lupus is the fatigue. The fatigue gets in the way of me enjoying my life with my children. The sunlight contributes to flare ups and fatigue. Therefore, I need to stay out of the sunlight, however, my girls play summer sports and love the beach and water parks. I show up for all their practices and games, but as soon as it is over, I am back home and in the bed. When it comes to the beach and water parks, I try to take them right before summer comes; and if the heat is too hot for me to bare, I take them in the fall. Although lupus is a big part of my life, I don't let it control my life. I like to say that I have lupus, lupus don't have me.

* * * *

Although I have lupus and lupus don't have me, lupus and PTSD are some of the main reasons why I homeschool my children. I can recall my children being in daycare and Pre-K and having to rush and hustle to get them to school on time. I mean, I would be a hot mess! I would be dropping the kids off with a bandana on and clothes from the night before… the same clothes from the day before. Literally looking like I was feeling… straight tired as hell!

I can recall, one day my child's teacher asked me if I was ok, and I cursed her out for asking me that dumb ass question. "Hell, naw I ain't ok, y'all start class too damn early and I am tired, hell are you ok??? Don't ask me no crazy shit like that no more, just take this baby!" So of course, she told the Director of the school that she thought something was wrong with me. So, then I had to check her (the Director) too.

Because of my PTSD, every time I had to drop my kids off at daycare I would be nervous and anxious beyond control. I am talking about hyperventilating and everything. Part of my PTSD is due to multiple sexual assaults against me. I just feared someone hurting my girls while I was away at work... or just not around period. I don't think I could have lived with myself if someone sexually, physically or verbally assaulted my babies. Which was why my children has had only one babysitter other than my niece. If my children were not with me, they were with their father.

Therefore, when I finally made the decision to homeschool, I knew I would not be looking back; and I haven't looked back either. However, I gotta tell ya, it has not been easy! With having a doctoral degree in education, I wanted to use my degree while homeschooling. I first tried Pre-K in my home and it didn't work out because I was tired as hell and kept falling asleep while trying to teach. It is one thing to fall asleep on your own kids, but it is another thing to fall asleep on someone else's child.

So, then I decided to open a tutoring center. However, the individual that was supposed to help me with the kids was unreliable and I ended up closing the center within six months of opening it.

Finally, I decided to teach online. However, that was tough too. The kids would always need my attention while I was trying to teach. So finally, I just said forget it! I went to apply for social security but I was denied because I was too educated not to be able to find employment… whatever the hell that means. And because I couldn't find work or I didn't know how to work as a single parent with two young children and a $100,000 student loan debt, I went into a deep depression.

The funny thing about me and depression is that I worked my hardest while going through depression. The work kept me from having to deal with my issues, problems and situations. I went all in on teaching my girls how to read and write and do math. Both of my children were reading and adding by the age of two… all because Mama was depressed. I was avoiding dealing with depression, so I threw myself into homeschooling my kids. I guess you can say that was my way of dealing.

However, don't get it twisted, it was not easy. The depression was deep and so real! The fatigue from the lupus was still whipping my ass, I was having daily migraines headaches and gaining weight like crazy because my joints were aching too bad to workout. More often than not, we did homeschooling from my bed. I would feel guilty and go out to join a homeschool co-operative group, only to get even more depressed, stressed and frustrated because I had to rush to get everyone out of the house and in class by 9:00 a.m. It was just too much.

Even though homeschool co-operatives were a bit too much on many days, I would still try to push through it because society has a way of making you feel like you are failing at homeschooling if you are not in a "socialization" group. But here is the thing, my children did not need a group to be socialized. In fact, they were over socialized. They were in gymnastics, ballet, music, art, playdates and camps with other kids. Hell, I even arranged community field trips to the police station and waste management plant. In fact, my children had a very fulfilled life.

Finally, after homeschooling for eight years and paying $1,200 for a homeschool co-operative group, I decided to release my guilt and shame and explained to my children that I had PTSD and lupus, and what that looks like for our family. They were 6 and 7 years old at that time. I then dropped out of the co-operative and decided to do homeschooling our way. What that means is that we have school in the bed when I don't feel well. If we are tired, we sleep in late. If I have doctor appointments, the girls go with me and bring their school work along. If we don't finish during the day, there is always the night and weekends. We don't stress with trying to get others to join us on a field trip; if we want to go on a field trip, we just jump in the car and go.

Yes, PTSD and lupus has had a major effect on my life, it contributed to the loss of my marriage and career and the onset of postpartum depression. Over the years, I have learned how to live life and homeschool while living with PTSD and lupus. Although it has been tough, I have been tougher.

Everyday life is a struggle, but everyone has a cross to bare, mine just happens to be PTSD and lupus. What don't kill you will make you stronger, right? On many days all I can do is praise God for the strength that He has bestowed upon me. And when that praise doesn't feel like enough, I praise God for allowing me to seek professional help before I threw the crying baby down the stairs. I praise God for the divorce, because it allowed me to see where my help truly comes from; Him and not from man. I praise God for choosing me to raise and educate my beautiful daughters. I praise God for continuing to pull me out of deep dark holes of depression. I praise God for patience and grace. And on any occasion, I praise God for saving me from the pit of hell.

Did you know?

There is an estimated 86.6% survival rate past 5 years of people diagnosed with **HODGKIN LYMPHOMA**.[4]

"Have a vision. Be demanding." - Colin Powell

~ CHAPTER FOUR ~

From The Inside Out, To The Outside In

BY LATRENDA CHIRELL BAILEY-RUSH, ED.S.

As I entered in the crowded room, I glanced over and saw a friend that I haven't seen in years. We began to hug and greet one another and started asking how things were going in each of our lives. The moment I said that I was recovering from cancer, she said those very words that I have yet to understand: "Girl, you don't look sick! As a matter of fact, I can't even tell you've been sick a day in your life!"

I took a step back and realized that sometimes people underestimate what life can do to people. Before you know it, the outside can affect the inside silently while the inside is suffering. Invisible chronic illness becomes an outer illness. My world is no longer normal and as soon as I share with someone what I am facing, they verbalize how I should look, which is a mirage of what is manifesting on the inside of me.

Little did people know that I have suffered from cancer, the diagnosis of Hodgkin's Lymphoma began to sink in with me. Day and night I thought about how I felt when the doctor gave the report of cancer. I could simply hear the doctor's voices conversing on the phone about me saying, "Her numbers are normal, but the biopsy says differently. She looks very healthy." I sank down in my spirit in sorrow of what am I to do.

I have four beautiful children and a loving husband. They need me. Cancer you don't belong in my life! Why did you come my way?

All types of questions swirled in my head. *How could this be? This has to be a dream. Not me! I exercise and eat healthy. This cannot be true. My God, do you think this report is a mix-up? I have to fight and get through this because my family needs me.*

Mental stability was going to be my biggest challenge. How am I to defeat those negative thoughts in the middle of the night? How can I disguise my sadness while I care for my children and remain vibrant for them? How to not throw a pity party and put on this façade for the outside world while screaming on the inside *why* and *help me*?

I sat in solitude feeling so very distant from everyone around me trying to contain my sanity and keep afloat. As times persisted, I had to grasp reality and come to grips with what was before me, take action and dig my heels in. During my treatments, my husband and I tried to keep things as normal as possible for our young children. Having two in diapers, one in Pre-K and our oldest daughter in second grade with no relatives nearby, things got tough and, at times, overwhelming for us all; so we decided to place scriptures on every wall, door, refrigerator, car and even our work office space.

I continued to teach despite the chemo treatments and pushed through the illness. I had coworkers that understood me (and some that didn't) and they would boldly ask, "Why are you here? Why won't you just go home? I don't think you should work right now."

My thoughts and expressions were not very nice because it frustrated me that they didn't understand. They were looking on the outside of my situation. There is a two-fold to inside out and the outside in, and that is mental health!

When one is battling a chronic illness, you fight with thoughts constantly, so you keep yourself busy to get your mind off of your true reality. And sometimes the inside rule the outside and things began to become visible and then verbal. I made up in my mind that once I could learn to control my thoughts, my feelings about the cancer would help me to begin living from the inside out which helped me to nourish myself from the outside in.

Everyday I meditated on one particular scripture in the Holy Bible and it truly helped me: II Corinthians 10:5-6 (King James Version), "Casting down imaginations, and every high thing that exalted itself against the knowledge of God, and bringing into captivity every thought to the obedience of Christ; And having in a readiness to revenge all disobedience, when your obedience is fulfilled."

My children suffered the most during my chemo treatments because they were not used to seeing me bald and always tired. That was terrible and scary. They were clingy and the separation anxiety increased. I remember having to part from my oldest daughter leaving her with one of my coworkers overnight because my daughter attended the same school. That next morning my surgery was schedule for 5:00 a.m., so I had no other choice but to leave her there overnight. It was the biggest decision I made but I knew she was in good hands. I am very grateful for my coworker that offered to help me, she took very good care of my daughter and made sure she was fed and well groomed for the next school day.

I went into my surgery feeling very sad and overwhelmed. I was looking forward to seeing all of my babies' faces after my surgery. It's a feeling no one could ever really describe, but it will bring you to the true appreciation of life, family and having your health.

* * * *

There are so many people in this world at some point in their lives that will face some type of illness or have to care for their loved one that are in need of care. Caring for a loved one can take on a major task and if you are not strong enough to take the bitter with the sweet, the journey will only lead to the road less taken. That road less taken is not always easy or popular either.

I have been so overwhelmed at times because the feeling inside makes you feel helpless. You are so used to moving around independently and then suddenly things change. I went from being able to bathe myself, to my husband bathing me. I went from barely standing and walking to the bathroom, to my husband literally carrying me to the toilet. It's a moment when wedding vows become 3-D!

I constantly say to myself the only thing that's constant is change! I watched my husband take care of our four children, change diapers, helping with homework and working a full-time job.

Caregivers are left juggling so many tasks and wearing so many hats just to make the world go around, until they will begin to feel overwhelmed themselves. So many people go unnoticed of how much help is really needed, from proper food preparation, household cleaning to basic lawn care. Caring for everyone but themselves takes a major toll.

The very moment I felt as though I was going to lose my mind was when my husband had to go through surgery and I had just finished treatments two days prior. I remember getting him home and comfortable and I finally got a chance to rest; then we both looked at each other and said, "Now who's going to take care of the babies?"

We both felt helpless! It was a moment where we had to create energy out of thin air. Only the good Lord above knows how we survived. I was thinking to myself, "What is really going on? What is the reason for this encounter?" I had no strength but the very thing that pushed me was the fact that my husband cared for me. Love can carry you through any situation! I found myself giving back in return what my husband selfishly gave to me.

I could only imagine what our children was feeling or even thinking, but I was determined to keep things as normal as possible and shower them with the love that they rightly deserved. Many people would only assume that everything was all right, but deep down inside we were in need of simple support.

Total strangers began out of nowhere helping us and giving us encouraging words to keep pushing. It is hard for people to understand what you are going through but it takes courage, love and selflessness in order to endure any illness.

I've learned that the two most important moments in a person's life is the day they are born and the day they find their purpose! I want to encourage others to never give up on yourself, never stop dreaming and don't push away help when you know you need it.

Be that helping hand to those that are in extreme need. Cook a meal, send a merry maid, and mow a lawn... every act of kindness matters. Always remember when someone gives of their time and energy to help one another, it will develop the heart from inside out to the outside in.

Did you know?

FIBROMYALGIA is not limited to age, even children can be diagnosed with the disease. Furthermore, people with lupus can also develop fibromyalgia.[5]

Romans 8:37 (King James Version), "Nay, in all these things we are more than conquerors through Him that loved us."

~ CHAPTER FIVE ~

See Me: Inner Pain, Outer Struggle

BY VYCE MOSES JOHNSON

The sneak attack was real. You know how you don't know danger is upon you until it snatches your purse and runs; or how you're walking along and step into a hole twisting your ankle, and just like that, your power walk is propped up by a metal crutch? You didn't set out to be mugged by some random, nor did you foresee yourself spending an evening in the emergency room getting a cast. When those unfortunate incidents occur, you may recover your stolen items or replace them, but you will heal and move on; your broken bone will mend and you'll be back to running or power walking with ease again, heal and move on. What happens, though, when the sneak attack occurs and you won't heal from it and you can't move on?

Chronic illness snatched my purse and ran, but I won't get that purse back. Chronic illness was that unexpected hole I stepped in, but the bones are crushed, diminished to a leisure walk, never to run again. What's agonizing is the fact that when I was attacked, so were those connected to me, but they failed to understand why I haven't healed and moved on. It is not my intention to give you lots of medical jargon, but to pull you into a life I didn't sign up for. This is my story of the inner pain and outer struggle of chronic illness. See me!

* * * *

In 2003, I was teaching at a middle school in Columbia, South Carolina when I felt like my arm weighed several extra pounds. I had never felt a heaviness like that nor the pain. It was on my right side. I started panicking, so they took me into the teacher's lounge and called the ambulance. My head was hurting as well, so they didn't want to take any chances that something serious was happening. After being seen at the emergency room, they determined that I was having a migraine and prescribed pain medicine.

Days turned to weeks and weeks to months, and I still wasn't feeling better. I still made at least another trip to the ER only to not have answers. I KNEW something was wrong with me. The final straw came when I felt like an elephant was sitting on my chest, so I had my husband take me to Doctor's Care. I tearfully explained what I had been experiencing—pain, fatigue, headaches, etc. The doctor did some examination and further questioning. I just wanted to know what was wrong and could I fix it. Finally, the best words, kinda, I had heard in over three months, "I know what's wrong with you." Yes! I knew something was wrong. I knew it wasn't just in my head. Those words brought instant relief, then took my breath away in the next moment.

Fibromyalgia... What is that?! According to the Mayo Clinic, "Fibromyalgia is a disorder characterized by widespread musculoskeletal pain accompanied by fatigue, sleep, memory and mood issues. Researchers believe that fibromyalgia amplifies painful sensations by affecting the way your brain processes pain signals."[6] Apparently, it wasn't life-threatening, but could and would disrupt quality of life.

Since 2003, my life has never been the same. This is largely in part because so many people had and/or have no clue what the condition is. Some believe it's a figment of our imagination. Clearly, you can't be in pain ALL the time. The fact of the matter is I most certainly am.

May 2006, I sat in a silent birthing room preparing to deliver a stillborn baby girl. The physical and mental pain was monstrous. The pain of pushing for nothing. The pain of fibromyalgia. The silent pain of hypertension that snatched my baby away—too much… simply unbelievable. Grief sent my fibro flares into another stratosphere. I couldn't stand. I couldn't breathe. I couldn't BE without pain!

I hurt with a love so strong, it sucked the wind from my soul. I cried until I was a shell of myself—weak and despondent. Everyone wanted me to be better because I was gonna make myself feel worse. I promise, I couldn't feel worse. *And who are YOU to tell ME how to feel?! Is YOUR kid dead? ARE THEY?!* Anger and despair fueled my chronic illness to a boiling point and wiped me out. The 'me' you saw then was a pile of nothingness. My fibromyalgia was so much worse being pregnant, but I endured because there was a greater purpose coming from the agony. When I lost my daughter, all I then carried was fibro coupled with pregnancy induced hypertension. I was in a dark place, and no one understood. No one could see me.

* * * *

I did become a mother when God built our family through adoption in 2007, but that presented a new web of challenges. Now, it's up and down stairs getting bottles, changing diapers, lifting and rocking a baby. The fibromyalgia was like, "What are you doing?!" I was over the moon excited to be a mother, but scared to death because this little life was in my hands and those hands were a little shaky. What do I do when I'm alone with my newborn and a pain flare takes me out? Did I mention stress causes flares? Yea... about that... In the midst of new motherhood and living with fibromyalgia, a new "one more thing" was headed to knock on my door. Could my life get any more complicated? The answer to that was: Absolutely!

Fast forward to 2008. I was referred to a rheumatologist for further blood work because I was otherwise healthy as far as the routine blood tests, but clearly something was brewing. Antinuclear antibodies (ANA) is a blood test that detects if the body is attacking itself. Diseases like lupus and rheumatoid arthritis are often diagnosed, in part, using this test to start. My results were positive yet inconclusive, meaning they did not point to any one particular autoimmune disorder, but I did have something.

The doctor named it 'undifferentiated connective tissue disease'. It could mimic several autoimmune illnesses and could manifest itself into a specific one later on. My 'specific' was discoid lupus which affects my skin, namely my eyelid. So now on top of chronic pain and fatigue, I also have an "ugly" eye—chronic illness sucks and I'm further lost. So, if you're keeping up, I have been diagnosed with fibromyalgia, hypertension and now an autoimmune illness.

What are you going to do? Do you want to take anything? Why don't you do this? Why don't you do that? You aren't trying to do anything for yourself.

In the years since I'd been diagnosed with fibromyalgia and an autoimmune disorder, I have heard these phrases from mostly family but also employers and onlookers who have no clue of the box I live in. I feel 100% trapped. The real me is hidden behind pain and aggravation. Again, I did NOT choose this! NONE of it!

Then to top it off, in walked depression. Trying to manage chronic illness on top of everything and everyone else, mental illness is definitely affected, or infected.

* * * *

There were ways to alleviate the pain and put a band-aid on the situation. Exercise, staying out of the sun or protecting yourself when you're outdoors, keeping stress levels to a minimum, blah blah blah. Often what helps, especially exercise, can exacerbate the problem, so you have to be careful not to overdo. Then, when you've worked all day moving around and such, the LAST thing you want to do is MORE moving, so I didn't.

I resolved myself to knowing this is how life was going to be, and depression set in. When it came and paid an unannounced visit to my life, it came with bags packed and a large storage container in the driveway to store its belongings. Tears, fears, doubts, and more tears. I laughed depressed. I worked depressed. I loved depressed. I was a mother depressed. I was chronically ill - DEPRESSED.

With this depression came weight gain... LOTS of weight gain. Not one condition I had, fibromyalgia, hypertension, autoimmune disease, could be helped with weight gain. I laid around feeling sorry for myself and packed on the pounds. I didn't care. I was numb but functioning, laughing, going places, but inside I was dying, unattractive, crying. The pain—physical and mental—were becoming too much to bear. I never once wanted to die, but I wasn't LIVING either. How did I allow my conditions to engulf my life like this? Why did this even happen to me? Deeper into the hole, I retreated.

I was looking for compassion and it was getting to be less and less. I got angry. WHY DON'T YOU CARE THAT I'M IN PAIN?! WHY WON'T YOU HELP ME?! STOP OFFERING ME MEDS AND SHOW ME SOME COMPASSION!

Behind the anger came more depression and retreating. I was in pain all the time to varying degrees. Fibromyalgia is not some sore muscle or a quick spasm. It lives and breathes with you. Undifferentiated connective tissue disease lives and breathes with you. The pain would be so great that I felt I couldn't stand, and that sent me into panic attacks. These panic attacks would have me visiting the ER or an immediate visit to the nearest doctor for care. These panic attacks would hold me hostage in the car, deathly afraid to go into work. My life was consumed with these problems and conditions and ailments. However, I am

NOT my conditions. The switch had to be flipped or I was going to lose my life.

* * * *

My feelings got hurt pretty bad. I had ballooned to over 300 pounds and someone very close to my heart hurt me to the core, but it was a wake up call. The person standing in the way of my wellness was me. The person who allowed things to get to this point was me. No one else's compassion; no one else's love; no one else's good intentions. Not my family; not my husband or parents; not my friends... ME.

I had accepted defeat. I wasn't trying to be better. So now, instead of the onlookers asking me what am I going to do, I had to ask myself that question. Nothing I was carrying meant death, so why was I accepting it as such? I spent the entire summer going to the gym. It was excruciating at first, but I got stronger. Was the pain gone? No, but I was now present in the fight and not getting knocked out every round. The weight started falling off, and as that occurred my will to go forward did also.

* * * *

Fibromyalgia is a what NOT a who. Undifferentiated connective tissue disease is a what NOT a who. For years, I allowed my conditions to define my life. Who am I when they are being managed? No. It's who I am whether in a flare or managed. Whether my eye is swollen shut or red rimmed from the discoid rash—I am still ME. I'm a mother, educator, writer, and tech savvy diva. I have been blessed to earn degrees battling chronic illness. I have written two books swinging and landing punches to chronic illness. I produced several plays while my body was under attack. I teach our future leaders and professionals even when I may have to take a few days to get my pain levels back to some normalcy. I say all that to say even though there are days when self-care is a must, I make a daily decision to LIVE beyond my conditions. I claimed my life back from the mugger who snatched my purse. I am recovering from the sneak attack.

I had to realize that my purpose was greater than my pain. I could choose to die to fibromyalgia and autoimmune disease or walk through it in triumph. God did not fashion me a loser. His word says in Romans 8:37 (King James Version), "Nay, in all these things we are more than conquerors through Him that loved us."

The chronic illnesses that plague me are in my makeup, but no longer do I stand in their shadow. They must stand in mine. I choose to thrive not just survive. I am present in my life now. On the days it seems chronic illness is winning, I remember that the fact I chose to get up means it already lost. I rest when I must, but I don't quit. The reflection I see and the reality you see is me, NOT my chronic illness.

Did you know?

It is estimated that 65 out of every 100,000 women and 12 out of every 100,000 men have primary biliary cholangitis, formerly known as **PRIMARY BILIARY CIRRHOSIS**.[7]

FIBROMYALGIA was once thought to be a mental disorder in the early 1800s. In 1976, the name of the condition was changed to "fibromyalgia" to further describe the symptom and tender points in the body.[8]

MIGRAINE is the third most prevalent illness in the world. In the U.S., it is reported that 18% of women, 6% of men, and 10% of children experience migraines.[9]

"Ensuring an optimistic future by empowering our legacies one voice and one community at a time." - Dr. Torre Brown

~ Chapter Six ~

Blessings Covered In Sh**

By Dr. Torre Brown, MABM, MSHRM, ThD, CLC, PC

I was what they called an "at-risk" teen growing up in St. Louis, Missouri. Raised in a low income single parent household, I struggled academically. Since I did not meet the standard of success set by the school system, the academic staff that was put in my life to help me succeed at the time were the ones that put negative obstacles in my way that hindered my success. They told my mom that I was not academically strong enough to go to college, and that I should instead either go to Vocational Technical School or seek a career instead.

My mother raised me that if you want to change something you must do something. If you want to make a positive change to your environment, you must go to college. So, though I didn't have the best grades and test scores, I was hungry for change.

The last thing I remember someone saying to me was, "When you come back to St. Louis, you bring back that Bachelors Degree they said you couldn't get." Little did they know, when I returned to St. Louis, I returned not only with my Bachelors Degree, but also with two Masters, my Doctorate, and three Certifications! Don't tell me God won't do it!

So, as you can see, I have always been a rebel with a cause. Destined to prove all naysayers wrong. At that point I became an advocate for change. A Game Changer. I changed the game where they said the game could not be changed by the players they said could not change the game. I tell people that I have the Harriet Tubman Syndrome. They told me I could get out, now I feel obligated to go back and save as many people as I can and show them that they can get out too.

December 28, 1998, two years into my marriage, my husband and I received a call from my Obstetrics and Gynecology (OB/GYN) doctor who asked me, "Do you want to have a baby today?" My answer was excitedly…. "YES!!!" She told me to head to the Birthing Center now.

It's game time! I was ready. I had been watching the T.V. Show *Baby Story* for eight months. I had everything baby and then some. Hubby and I were ready. Only thing missing was baby girl, Tyler Denise.

Long story short, I was induced because I never dilated past three centimeters after 16 hours in labor. I was stuck in the back six times with the epidural, which only numb the left side of my back. So, when they decided to do a Cesarean, or C-Section, I had to have a Spinal Tap—yes getting one final shot in my back, making that a total of seven shots in my spine.

I was numb all the way up to my throat. I literally could not feel myself breathe. I thought I was going to die. I did not think I was going to live to see my baby girl even take her first breath here on earth.

The next day, on December 29th at 7:28 p.m., Tyler Denise Anderson Brown made her entrance into the world, and yes you guessed it, covered in sh**. Hers of course, and maybe a little of mine, but that's another story for another chapter—maybe geriatrics or something (smile)... back to my greatest accomplishment in the world thus far: my blessed angel, Tyler.

Now I am still on the surgical table wide open with all of my organs laid out waiting to be placed back inside, while I wondered if I was going to live long enough to hold my precious angel. I looked over at my husband holding Tyler in his arms as I was slowly losing consciousness and struggled to breathe. I remember that I kept willing myself to keep my eye on my prize, which was my daughter, Tyler. My new reason to live.

After the surgeon pieced me back together and rolled me out to my room. Still struggling to keep my eyes open, I could barely see my family's faces. I could hear sounds of excitement from seeing the baby but then quickly turned to shock as they watched me following behind in Intensive Care highly sedated. It would be a few days before I would truly be able to see and hold Tyler. Many family comedic stories still exist from those five days in the hospital.

I was finally released from the hospital only to return the following day due to a terrible headache. Come to find out that during the seventh spinal tap injection while I was in labor, my spinal column was punctured and was leaking spinal fluid. That was the reason for the excruciating headaches whenever I sat up or walked. The cure was to take blood from a vein and inject it in the spinal column again, my eighth injection in the back, which would cause a blood clot that would close the hole leaking the spinal fluid. Pain would be alleviated after laying flat on my back for six hours straight.

My husband, my high school sweetheart (a United States Navy Man) just had a healthy, beautiful baby girl. There were only three problems. Let me explain.

* * * *

I felt as if I was babysitting. "Where are the parents of this child?" I thought to myself. I loved my baby, but because my own recovery took so long, it took up to three months before really bonding with my angel. Plus, she had colic and was crying all the time. I was extremely sleep deprived, like most new moms.

"I think I may need to talk to an attorney because I have been hoodwinked, tricked, fooled, made a mockery!" I thought to myself. I mean, I watched that damn *Baby Story* television show for eight months during my pregnancy, and my story was nothing like what I saw on that show.

There was nothing cute about my story at all. Now, don't get me wrong, there was some love at first sight. When I first saw that morphine bottle (also known as Tyler) for the first time, I fell helplessly and hopelessly in love for the next five days. That's how long my initial love was for my miracle baby. Just being honest.

You must understand. Literally, my liver and spleen were in my throat. I had been stuck in my spine a total of seven times only to be numb on half of my body for sixteen full hours of labor. I was rolled out into Intensive Care, not with full makeup or family photo shoot at the park like I saw on that show. That was no cute *TLC Baby Story*. They would never show my story on *Baby Story*. I tell you what though, *Baby Story* should give a disclaimer that your story may experience hell and may not be the beautiful lies the stories aired on their network. That's all I'm saying. I was set up from the beginning for failure.

* * * *

Now this was the big one. What started off as the "baby blues" is medically known as postpartum depression, which affects 80% of new mothers. So my story goes like this all of sudden, I used to just cry, get upset and stressed out all the time for no reason.

Well, I guess I did have a reason. I had a new baby that never slept. All she did was eat, cried, screamed and pooped. Oh, and she vomited. I mean she used to projectile vomit like the exorcists. I literally waited for her head to spin in circles. At which point I would call my Pastor because I was outta there! Jesus could have her! That's what I used to say.

Along with all of those rolling emotions, I remember feeling helpless and wanting to die like all the time. I remember one day in particular riding in the car with my husband and wanting to just open the passenger door and fall out.

One night when I couldn't get the baby to stop crying, I remember calling my mom and saying that I was going to jump off the third floor balcony because I couldn't take it anymore. The anxiety was too much to handle. I was having panic attacks and didn't even know it.

Now mind you, never during this time did I ever think of harming the baby. I loved Tyler. It was all me. I blamed me. I thought I was weak. A failure. I watched my mom, grandmother and aunts do this single handedly with multiple children and here I was failing with just one child. I was a disgrace.

When I went to the doctors, I resisted help. I thought they were crazy. I'm a black woman. I was raised to be prepared to live a hard life. This was what I had been training for all my life. This was just 'game' time. I was 'culturally disillusioned' and 'improperly programmed.'

Okay, now I know I can't just drop culturally disillusioned on you and not explain. I say culturally disillusioned because, in the African American culture, we are created to be strong, never ask for help or handouts unless you are finally admitting that all those past statements are true and you are a failure.

At that point my doctor was recommending daily mental health medication treatment and bi-weekly therapy. And my response was very naturally, "Oh hell naw!! First of all, crazy people take medication and I'm not crazy. Secondly, go to counseling? Where they do that at?"

I was also "improperly programmed" that you don't discuss your struggles with strangers. I bet every person reading this can relate to or have heard these statements at least once in your lifetime:

"Never talk or trust strangers."

"Don't be telling my business to nobody."

"What goes on in this house, stays in this house."

"Don't be airing our dirty laundry out there in these streets."

"Don't let me hear about my business or house out in these streets."

"All you need is Jesus."

If you can relate to any variations of those 'sayings in the Black household', then you too may have been programmed. We called it 'being raised' at the time but me, now all grown up and with my very expensively priced multiple degrees, I recognize I was programmed and disillusioned. The reality being: I was NOT a failure and it was okay to ask for help.

Growing up in a Christian household and loving God, I was pushed further from the church during the darkest time of my life by the very people that were supposed to bring me closer to God. I mean, seriously, the things I were told by the church were:

"All you need is Jesus."

"Those feelings of depression is just the devil."

"You just need to pray more."

"You just need to read the Bible more."

"Anxiety is just you trying to resist the Holy Spirit."

"When you feel like you having an anxiety attack you need to read the Bible."

"You need to fast more."

"God don't need no medication to help Him."

"You have to have more faith that God can heal you."

"Why you claiming it?"

"There's no such thing as depression!"

"God helps those who helps themselves."

"Stop having a pity party!"

Yeah, the church had a WHOLE lot to say about my condition! So as you can imagine, I didn't get a lot of help from the church. Instead, the devil used this time to try to claim me as his victory, but it was my true love for God and my knowledge of Him and His word that again let God keep me as His.

* * * *

I didn't understand how I did the most natural thing in the world for a woman to do (to bring forth life) and that same thing devastated my life. Having my first daughter in 1998 changed my life forever in many ways. She was my greatest accomplishment at the time. She was my angel and reason for living. Yet the process of bringing her into the world almost ended my life, and a week later, from postpartum, I wanted to take my own life. I was fighting a physical turned mental war. But because of Tyler, I didn't carry out the suicidal thoughts that were running wild in my mind.

On March 8, 2000, I took another devastating blow: I lost my dad. That was a blow I thought I never knew how to come up from. I laid in the bed unable to physically get up.

Asking God for instruction on how to rise. I heard no words. I laid there helpless for hours. Then I heard two-year-old Tyler crying through the baby monitor.

With no one home but only the two of us, her dad was deployed overseas, we were all each other had. So, I got up for her and I had been getting up for her ever since. As you can see, Tyler was my angel. My life saver. She was sent to get me through that rough time. Had I not had her, I would have given up a long time ago. I felt like I had no reason to continue living until she came along.

In 2007, seven years after that great depression, I gave birth to my second angel, Trinity, whom I named after the Holy Trinity. And in all her glory, whatever her beautiful older sister did not destroy on her entry into the world, Trinity took care of upon her arrival! Yep, another hard delivery!

Now, imagine telling a young black woman who was told that she was un-educatable after she finally earned her Bachelors, two Masters, a Doctorates and two Certifications that she could no longer work! After all of that fighting to get those degrees, I was now faced with having to stop working and apply for disability after having two children. Another kick to my stomach. I was devastated yet again. I couldn't believe that was happening to me, an independent woman that God created and my mother raised me to be.

Here's another fact: more than 42.5 million Americans are living with mental illness at the time of this book. And that's just what has been reported.

Sometimes, just waking up in the morning was a disappointment to me and too painful to bare. Sometimes I even thought it became God's little joke that He continued to wake me up to the same roller coaster feelings of despair and helplessness, which seemed to be an endless tunnel of darkness.

* * * *

So, like Harriet Tubman, allow me to take you to true Peaceful Freedom. Peaceful Freedom is a freedom not from pain or discomfort, but a freedom of peace of mind and knowing that this is all just temporary for the time being until you are called to a place of true Heavenly Freedom. I'm not going to sugar coat things and say that every day is a good day. They say you take things one day at a time. I say that I take it one minute at a time, because an entire day is sometimes too much.

You take one step forward and two steps back sometimes. When it comes to the ailments that I live with many lose their battles every minute, sometimes seconds, of the day. So, each minute I'm still breathing is a blessing and I'm winning.

No matter how helpless you feel. No matter how far you have come, there's still room to move. Even if you take two steps forward and three steps back. At least you're still taking steps. There is someone out there that can no longer step. The battle is not over until it is over and even then, there is still victory when you reap your true rewards in your afterlife.

I am a Warrior. A Rebel with a Cause. I refuse to take this lying down. Together we are unstoppable. I am a movement by myself, but we are a force together.

* * * *

I only get one chapter in this book, but you best believe the story goes on. What I can say, there was light at the end of that tunnel. Even though I continue to live with multiple alignments consisting of fibromyalgia, chronic migraines, and primary biliary cirrhosis, my alignments don't define me, I define them. I'm an advocate for life not a victim. I make it my goal to research, educate and advocate.

It is my divine purpose to touch a life every day. I am just trying to live everyday as if it is my last, with no regrets, with my family and friends. I have two beautiful "Angel Legacies", Tyler and Trinity, who are making me super-duper proud every day. There are days I want to give up, but I can't, because of my two legacies, it's because of them I can.

Never in my wildest dreams did I think the most normal thing in the world for a woman to do would change my life so drastically. I knew giving birth would be so good, but I never thought it would be tragic.

If it was not for my grandmother, mom and sister who told me 'yes', when everyone else told me 'no', I would have given up a long time ago. They were my foundation and taught me everything I know. I followed their footsteps until I was able to walk on my own.

I thank my Mom so much for raising me and my sister so well, and installing such a deep love and faith in God that I was able to recognize that God so loved us that He gave His only Son for our sins and salvation. A God that would do *that* would come to give us many blessings in many forms, disguises, means and for many reasons.

So, go figure. Why would He not give me two beautiful, petite, perfectly designed blessings covered in sh**? Granted, it is because of childbirth I damn near feel like I'm dying every day. Even though they both came into the world covered in sh**, they are still the best blessings in the world a mother could ever receive.

Did you know?

To date, almost 10 million Americans have been diagnosed with **FIBROMYALGIA**; and there is no known cure for this chronic illness.[10] Instead, treatment for fibromyalgia includes proper self-care to reduce painful symptoms associated with the illness.[11]

"My mission in life is not merely to survive, but to thrive; and to do so with some passion, some compassion, some humor, and some style." - Maya Angelou

~ Chapter Seven ~

Living with Fibromyalgia

By Gretchen Hyatt

I can tell you that I have had a chronic illness my whole life. I don't remember ever *not* having it or being affected by it. When it was first presented to me, it was presented in the form of a nervous stomach. It was presented to me as I was being disobedient and getting beaten for how the triggers would make me act. I hate thinking about my life when I was little because those triggers that I couldn't identify at that time made my life a living hell.

Those triggers made people look at me a certain way that I was not; and it made people treat me a certain way. It forever changed how I look at life, how I look at people, how I look at relationships, how I want to be around people, how I want to raise my kids, where I want to live, how I think, how I eat, how I look at myself, how I look at my body, how I present myself, how I deal with things, how I compartmentalize things. It's just a cycle, a snowball effect.

If that one 'thing' could have been properly diagnosed, or educated to me and my family... if somebody would have just explained to me and my parents why I reacted the way I did... then maybe I could look back on my childhood and think more good than bad. Then maybe I wouldn't be running from writing this book, running from facing my pain, running from the bigger things I could be doing with my life.

Instead, it's a thorn. It's a thorn in my life and no matter how perfect I try to be, it always pop back up and turn my life upside down. Again, my story started when I was a kid having panic attacks. I don't remember not ever having this anxiety in my life. It's just now I know what 'it' was all these years later.

* * * *

It's amazing how things begin to make sense as you're older. Looking back now as an adult, I can identify the triggers. Like whenever somebody regurgitated, it would make me shake to the point where I would run out of the room with my heart beating out of my chest. I couldn't speak, I just ran away and I felt like somebody was trying to kill me. I couldn't explain this to my family. I couldn't explain this to people who saw me react like this. To them, I was a freak. I was disobedient. I was putting myself in danger and I was made fun of, and I was beaten severely countless of times. It made me not want to go places, afraid to be around sick people.

The memories that I have growing up were only good when I was alone. They were only good when I could control the environment, usually by lying or manipulating a situation. That's when I could have control over the anxiety. Not understanding the 'why' and not being able to put it into words, not being able to control how I reacted to the triggers… all of that kept me in bondage my whole life.

* * * *

My grandmother died when I was 15-years-old and a part of me died with her. She was the only one who made me feel accepted, needed or wanted. At that time, with everything going on, I coped with her passing by getting involved with boys and sex, and lots of it. I just didn't care anymore. I started skipping school for these boys. For some strange reason, I felt more comfortable with them. I knew they didn't care about me, and truth be told, I didn't care about myself. I just needed a space to escape my own thoughts and my own pain. And I didn't have to tell them my secret. They didn't care as long as I was putting out, it didn't matter. It was the perfect cocktail.

When I went to college, I figured out that if I had a real cocktail and was buzzed, my nerves would calm down, I would feel better and I could be around people without running into bathroom stalls and crying my eyes out. It was under the influence that I felt free. So that's how I managed my life with anxiety, through drinking often, especially at events where there were a lot of people.

Drinking and partying became my norm of dealing with the anxiety of large crowds and sick people. As a matter of fact, I never wanted kids because I knew they would get sick and I wouldn't be able to handle that or control the triggers. Not the way I was. Though, funny enough, I always wanted to be married. I couldn't imagine my life not having someone in it. I just did not want to be a mother.

But, as life would have it, I had gotten pregnant and the father of my child threatened to leave me if I aborted her. I loved him, so I kept the baby. Losing him was far more dire to me than aborting her. But I was so afraid of her. There were times when she was sick and I couldn't care for her because of the triggers, and my parents and her dad had to step in. I couldn't care for her when she was sick. My mind and my nerves wouldn't allow it.

* * * *

After my divorce from her dad, I got a good job and went back to school. My life seemed to be perfect according to normal standards of perfect. And then I started to get extremely depressed to the point of suicidal ideation (in other words, I was having suicidal thoughts). I kept telling my doctor something wasn't right and they kept sending me to a therapist. Then finally, my doctor put me on some medicine that made me have a psychotic episode. I ended up in the hospital and was diagnosed with a mental illness, manic depression actually. It was Type 2 at first, but then because of how reactive from the antidepressants, they changed it to Type 1 manic depression. It was with this diagnosis that I gained a sense of clarity, like everything felt back to normal.

I was put on a strong medication regimen, told to go to therapy and see my psychiatrist once a month. A part of me didn't want to accept this. At first I thought, 'Okay, great. I wasn't wrong. There was something wrong with me.' But then, on the other hand I thought, 'Well, it can't be a mental illness because then it is going to make me look like a freak.' Mind you, I was dealing with anxiety that happened randomly when someone would throw up in front of me. Little did I know that the anxiety and the manic depression triggered each other. Consequently, I had countless trips to the hospital. I was fine as long as I was taking my medication; but then when I felt better, I didn't think I needed the medication. When I was off my meds, the psychotic episodes would happen and I would spiral out of control, ending up back in the hospital. It was like a revolving door.

This continued on for two years, then in 2005, I met the guy of my dreams! He was a military man that wanted to marry me and take me and my daughter to London, where he was going to be stationed. I worked very hard to get myself stable so that I could be a good wife for him. I got passports for me and my daughter, then told my parents. They weren't in agreement with my decision. They thought I was moving too fast, but my mind was made up.

Maybe three weeks before me and my daughter were to leave for London to be with my fiancé, he sent me an email telling me that he didn't want me because I already had a daughter. I remember going numb, I was devastated. I started working out to cope with my heart break. I stopped eating, lost my appetite. I just put myself into work and sex with random dudes just to distract myself from the pain.

One day a coworker had a stomach virus and had given it to everybody in the office. I got sick too, but even after I got over the stomach virus, I would have panic attacks every time I had to go in to work. I would literally feel like I had to throw up and would have to leave the office. The attacks were so intense that I ended up having to quit that job and got another one. The same thing happened again at the new job, so I just kept moving from one job to another. I couldn't work and ended up back in the hospital because I lost a whole lot of weight from not eating, plus I was having psychotic episodes. Life was so bad for me during that time. I couldn't tell if I was really sick or if it was all in my head. I was miserable.

* * * *

A little over a year after being diagnosed with manic depression, my life took another turn. One evening my coworker and I went to the sports bar next door to the bank where we worked. I knew mixing alcohol with my psychiatric medicine was against the doctor's orders, but I didn't listen. After a night of heavy drinking while on my meds, I remember going to work the next day feeling like I was coming down with the flu. I was running a fever and I was told to go home early.

I went to my mom's house to sleep but when I tried to get out of the bed to use the bathroom, I fell straight to the floor. I was in so much pain, I couldn't move and my mother couldn't get me up either. I called a friend to take me to the emergency room and was immediately admitted to the hospital in critical condition. Apparently I had developed rhabdomyolysis, a virus that destroys your muscle tissue and puts dead muscle fibers into your bloodstream, which is very poisonous. I was on the verge of kidney failure and the doctors were doing everything they could to bring me out of it. Had I not gone to the emergency room when I had, I would've died. I was informed by my doctor that it would take a while for me to recover fully from this virus that sent me into renal (kidney) failure causing muscle damage throughout 90% of my body.

I was in the hospital so long that I lost my job at the bank. And basically, I just focused on recovery and school. Just the dynamics of all of that, my body was never the same and I was then diagnosed with fibromyalgia, a chronic illness which is an overactive nerve condition that causes extreme muscle pain. So it's like, again, this 'thing' has taken over my life, and I am both mentally and physically f*cked! There's no sweet way to put it. My way of coping with it all (the drinking, partying, sexing) was not the best way of coping with it at all and actually ended up making matters worse. All I knew was this balancing act of living with a mental and physical chronic illness was exhausting.

* * * *

I spent the next three years taking pain meds to get through the day with no pain, drinking caffeine to stay awake and have energy, and having to explain to people all the time why I couldn't show up for events anymore, why I was losing weight, and why I didn't want people to touch me.

I would love to say that my life with fibromyalgia has gotten easier over time, however, it just seems like more parts of my body has become impacted by this illness which caused me to have to create new modifications. It is becoming increasingly more difficult for me to type on my laptop, or swipe my cell phone to communicate with people via text message, or to post things on social media. My finger tips are extremely inflamed and it feels like carpet burns. I have found it very useful to use the talk-to-text feature on all of my devices whenever possible. There are days that I still cannot walk or apply pressure to my legs or arms.

I'm extra grateful when I'm not waking up from a panic attack. Life since all of the diagnoses is filled with lots of doctors appointments, medications and adjustments to medications, figuring out what can I change, such as diet, exercise and therapy. You know, trying to relinquish as much stress as possible. I've found that during this journey, a lot of my triggers are coming from stress, food choices, lack of exercise, or lack of sleep. So once those things are adjusted, it helps along with medication. I've also discovered that hot bath soaks with lavender or eucalyptuses oil helps a lot too.

As far as the anxiety, what has helped me is identifying subconsciously all of my triggers and finally dealing with them. Going through a 12-step program for alcoholism helped me as well. Sobriety played a huge role in pulling out a lot of my hurts and fears by providing a safe space for me to talk about them, getting some answers, and getting some type of closure or resolution on them. They became less and less triggering in my life.

* * * *

My everyday life today looks like this: I am currently separated from my second husband. I have three children: an infant, a toddler, and a young adult. My days are still filled with doctors' appointments (both me and my children). Along with single-handedly raising my young babies, I still have to keep up with my therapy appointments, med management, work full-time as well as attend support meetings for the alcohol and the anxiety. I'm actually a leader in the recovery program.

My life is nothing what I thought it was going to be. Things were so bad that I thought the best that I would ever be able to be in life was bedridden, collecting a social security and disability check. I wouldn't be able to travel, or have children, or even work again. That's not my life. I fought hard to get a footing or a handle on these diagnoses. I dreamed a lot while I was bedridden, recovering from the Rhabdo virus. I dreamed of driving and seeing trees and mountains and valleys and water, and it would make me so happy. I held on to those dreams and those visions because I just knew one day that would be me. That's what made me fight because I wanted to actually see that.

And it finally happened in 2012 through our drive through West Virginia… the vision that I had from 2004 was right before me. That was my vision. That's what helped me rehabilitate and get to a place where I could walk and function on my own without any help. So I would tell anyone, no matter how bleak your situation looks, hold on to those moments, those dreams, and let that be your strength. Truth be told, I don't know what my life is going to be like day-to-day. I just cherish the little moments and I try not to beat myself up on the big things I can't do.

There are certain days I can't pump my gas. There are certain days I can't take my trash out. There are certain days I can't do my laundry. There are certain days I can't cook because I can't stand the smell of food. I have to keep the food basic for my kids. It's crazy but then again, that's my new normal. That's my life.

The best advice I can give you is to talk to as many doctors that are experts in your condition as possible. I actually ended up finding a fibromyalgia specialist when I moved to Charlotte, North Carolina, and that doctor gave me the best treatment plan possible, which helped me get the fibromyalgia somewhat under control. I still can't control days where the weather doesn't work in my favor, but there are other things that, you know, at least I know what the contributing factors are and the things that I can work on.

And I have to give myself permission to cry, to scream, to yell, to curse, to *not* do, to *not* deal, to *not* stay in those moments… I give myself permission to do everything I need to do. I affirm it. That's so important to do because sometimes we feel like because of where we are, or who we are, or how we were raised, or how we were blessed, that we can't give ourselves permission to not be perfect in an imperfect world. But I try to stay a realist.

Being transparent has also been a big help. I don't glaze over what's really going on. No matter how traumatic, no matter how painful, no matter if I overindulged in food or a little too much sex, no matter if I stayed in the bed a little too long, if I cuddled with my kids just a little bit too long, if I lied and told them I'll be out of the bathroom in about five minutes when I was going to be there for 15 minutes… I mean, I stay in a place of *real*.

I had to create a new natural support system for myself. Don't let anything detour you from making moves that are going to be healthier for you. For me, a warmer climate is always healthier. I absolutely love living on the water. It gives me a better sense of balance and it just does something that makes me feel good. So I would tell you, if it's healthy, safe, ethical or moral, legal, and even if it's outside the box, do what works best for you. This is your recovery and your recovery is not going to look like mine or anybody else's. Trust the journey.

~ The End ~

About the Pioneer Author

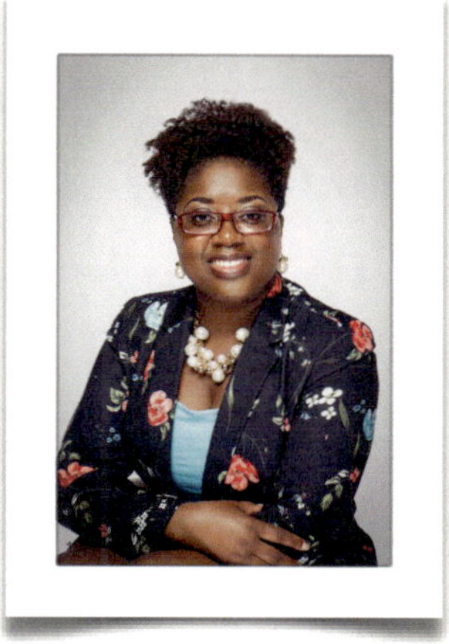

Dr. Marquita S. Blades is an award-winning Educator, international speaker, author, and education consultant with 16 years of experience as a high school science teacher and manager of national Science, Technology, Engineering and Math (STEM) programs for high-achieving high school students. During her time working with public school districts, she also served as a curriculum & assessment developer and professional learning facilitator for multiple school districts in the metropolitan Atlanta area.

Dr. Blades is currently a full-time Education Consultant, the owner of Dr. Blades Consulting, and the host of The Dr. Marquita Blades Show-Candid Conversations that Create Change, a radio show dedicated to discussing current trends and issues in education. Dr. Blades' Consulting firm offers solutions to learning institutions and individuals through professional development programs, curriculum and assessment development, and conference development and programming services. Dr. Blades is also the founder of The Mediocre Teacher Project© which helps other teachers avoid and battle through burnout by incorporating their unique gifts and talents into their daily practice. Dr. Blades has presented at numerous conferences including the International Academic Forum, International Conference on Innovation in Science Education, and the Innovative Schools Summit.

Dr. Blades earned a Bachelor of Interdisciplinary Studies in Broad Field Science from Georgia State University, a Master of Science in Technical and Professional Communication from Southern Polytechnic State University, and a Doctor of Education in Instructional Leadership from Nova Southeastern University. When she is not working, Dr. Blades enjoys reading, cooking, and traveling with her husband.

For more information, you can visit Dr. Blades' website: www.drmarquitablades.com

Follow her on Social Media:

Facebook: Dr. Blades Consulting

Twitter: @DrMBlades

LinkedIn: Dr. Marquita Smith Blades

Footnotes

[1]. The National Resource Center on Lupus. (2018). Lupus facts and statistics. Retrieved from https://resources.lupus.org/entry/facts-and-statistics

[2]. Sirven, Joseph I., MD and Shafer, Patricia O., RN MN. (2014, March 14). Facts about Seizures and Epilepsy. Retrieved from https://www.epilepsy.com/learn/about-epilepsy-basics/facts-about-seizures-and-epilepsy

[3]. The National Resource Center on Lupus. (2018). Lupus facts and statistics. Retrieved from https://resources.lupus.org/entry/facts-and-statistics

[4]. National Cancer Institute. (2008-2014). Cancer stat facts: Hodgkin lymphoma. Retrieved from https://seer.cancer.gov/statfacts/html/hodg.html

[5]. Centers for Disease Control and Prevention. (2018, April 3). Fibromyalgia. Retrieved from https://www.cdc.gov/arthritis/basics/fibromyalgia.htm

[6] Mayo Foundation for Medical Education and Research. (2018). Fibromyalgia. Retrieved from https://www.mayoclinic.org/diseases-conditions/fibromyalgia/symptoms-causes/syc-20354780

[7]. The National Institute of Diabetes and Digestive and Kidney Diseases Health Information Center. (2017, March). Definition & facts of primary biliary cholangitis (primary biliary cirrhosis). Retrieved from https://www.niddk.nih.gov/health-information/liver-disease/primary-biliary-cholangitis/definition-facts

[8]. Pfizer Inc. (2016). Fibrocenter's History of Fibromyalgia. Retrieved from https://www.fibrocenter.com/fibromyalgia-disease

[9]. Migraine Research Foundation. (2018). About migraines. Retrieved from http://migraineresearchfoundation.org/about-migraine/migraine-facts/

[10]. National Fibromyalgia & Chronic Pain Association. (2014). Fact sheet. Retrieved from https://www.fmcpaware.org/fibromyalgia/fm-fact-sheet.html

[11]. American College of Rheumatology. (2018). Fibromyalgia. Retrieved from https://www.rheumatology.org/I-Am-A/Patient-Caregiver/Diseases-Conditions/Fibromyalgia

Made in the USA
Monee, IL
05 November 2026

67383129R00076